Open Your

For Beginners

HOW TO AWAKEN YOUR THIRD EYE AND DECALCI-FY YOUR PINEAL GLAND

Written By

Mia Rose

☐ Copyright 2019 by Mia Rose - All rights reserved.

This document is geared towards providing exact and reliable information in regards to the topic and issue covered. The publication is sold with the idea that the publisher is not required to render accounting, officially permitted, or otherwise, qualified services. If advice is necessary, legal or professional, a practiced individual in the profession should be ordered.

- From a Declaration of Principles which was accepted and approved equally by a Committee of the American Bar Association and a Committee of Publishers and Associations.

In no way is it legal to reproduce, duplicate, or transmit any part of this document in either electronic means or in printed format. Recording of this publication is strictly prohibited and any storage of this document is not allowed unless with written permission from the publisher. All rights reserved.

The information provided herein is stated to be truthful and consistent, in that any liability, in terms of inattention or otherwise, by any usage or abuse of any policies, processes, or directions contained within is the solitary and utter responsibility of the recipient reader. Under no circumstances will any legal responsibility or blame be held against the publisher for any reparation, damages, or monetary loss due to the information herein, either directly or indirectly.

Respective authors own all copyrights not held by the publisher.

The information herein is offered for informational purposes solely, and is universal as so. The presentation of the information is without contract or any type of guarantee assurance.

The trademarks that are used are without any consent, and the publication of the trademark is without permission or backing by the trademark owner. All trademarks and brands within this book are for clarifying purposes only and are the owned by the owners themselves, not affiliated with this document.

Contents

Introduction

I want to thank you and congratulate you for getting the book, "Open Your Third Eye, For Beginners".

This book contains proven steps and strategies on how to de-calcify your Pineal Gland and open your Third Eye.

The book explores the facts, as far as they are known, the history and misconceptions in relation to this amazing subject. It provides a good, simple and practical set of steps to enable you to open your Third Eye and begin to benefit from the practical and spiritual advantages that this will open up to you. The book is designed to be a no-nonsense approach that anybody can implement and one which will give you all the tools you need to explore the world with your eyes, all three of them, wide open! Covering practical steps to de-calcify your Pineal Gland, meditation and crystal healing techniques to activate your Third Eye, along with what to expect once you have done so, the book provides a single resource for those new to both the concept and practice of Third Eye techniques.

Thanks again for reading this book, I hope you enjoy it!

Chapter 1: More to the Third Eye Than Meets the Eye

You may have heard of the "Third Eye" but not be clear on what it is, or how it functions. It may be that you've heard of it vaguely in relation to some strange, mysterious and wildly New Age ideas! The Pineal Gland, on the other hand is less well known but both the Third Eye and the Pineal Gland are closely related.

In terms of the Third Eye itself you may have some concept that it's connected either to Eastern mystical traditions or, in Western Culture, to clairvoyant abilities and/or in connection with seeing the dead. These concepts are, to some extent, founded on fact but there is much more to the Third Eye than, well, meets the eye! This book explores the subject for those who know a very little about the subject and would like to know more.

The concept of the Third Eye is not simply about clairvoyance or the ability to see and communicate with the dead – it's a far deeper spiritual and mystical concept. In many traditions, the Third Eye relates to our ability to connect to the greater powers in the universe and to deeply connect with our own inner self. The French philosopher, Rene Descartes, devoted much study to the concept of the Third Eye and, in particular, its relation to the Pineal Gland (more on this shortly). Descartes described this gland as the "seat of the soul".

In Eastern traditions, particularly Hinduism and Buddhism, a great emphasis was placed on this third, invisible eye. It is identified as one of the major energy points of the human body and is located on the forehead above the eyes. The energy centers are referred to as the Chakras and this particular Chakra is identified as the "brow Chakra" ("Ajna" to give it its traditional name. Opening, or becoming aware of the brow chakra, in these traditions is considered essential for human development, for the evolution of the soul and in the quest for ultimate enlightenment. In Western traditions the Third Eye is considered to be located in the Pineal Gland itself, which is located in the brain, roughly in the same location as the brow Chakra but a little deeper below the skin.

What Is the Pineal Gland?

The Pineal Gland is found in several mammals and also in several reptile species. In the latter, the term Third Eye is more obviously accurate. The gland is located on the surface of the brain and, in some species, protrudes visibly from the skin, forming a literal Third Eye, slightly above and between the usual two. The gland is sensitive to light, although it cannot see images. In the human body the Pineal Gland is peculiar in several respects. Considered a "vestigial" organ in some species (one that evolved for a reason but, although remaining, has become obsolete) the Pineal Gland in humans retains some important functions.

The gland is the only structure in the human brain which sits on the "mid-line" (simply the center of the brain) and does not have another half. The majority of the brain is formed in a mirror image – i.e. the two "hemispheres" which you may be familiar with. The fact that this gland sits centrally and appears to link the two sides of the brain is one of the main reasons that it is identified with abilities that include intuition and clairvoyance. As in other species, the Pineal Gland retains a photo-sensitive quality (sensitive to light) and it is responsible for the production of melatonin. This hormone derives from serotonin and is partly responsible for moderating mood (in a good way) and has an important function in relation to modulating sleep patterns (both daily and seasonally). Finally, the Pineal Gland is different to other areas of the brain in that it is directly linked to the rest of the body through the blood stream. The brain is protected by a membrane known as the "brain-blood-barrier". This "filter" stops toxins affecting the brain to avoid infections – these are extremely rare in the brain as a result. This unique quality makes the Pineal Gland both part of the brain and the body in a way that is not the case with other parts of the brain itself. The blood flow that it receives is the second highest in the body, second only to the kidney.

One significant effect of this connection of the Pineal Gland to the rest of the body is that it is an area that is susceptible to the process of "calcification"; this is the process by which calcium salts are deposited in soft tissue, causing them to harden. This is a natural process that occurs with aging but in the case of the Pineal Gland it seems to develop more rapidly than in other parts of the body and has been noted in children as young as two and is common in roughly half the population by the later teens. This calcification process is one reason that many people believe that the Pineal Gland loses function quickly in most individuals and, as we'll see later in the book, a possible cause for the intuitive and clairvoyant skills that we all naturally possess being limited in many people today.

Chapter 2: The Third Eye; Background and History

The term the "Third Eye" is a relatively modern one – which explains a lot of those New Age associations that the term may bring to mind. However, the idea behind the concept is a very old one indeed and references can be found relating to the idea right back to our ancestor's earliest days – across most imaginable or recorded civilizations. In most traditions, the Third Eye was considered a symbol of enlightenment and closely linked with belief that it is possible to transcend physical sensations and the boundaries that they impose on our perception of the world.

References can be found to the concept of the Third Eye across many cultures. In ancient China it was better known as the "Mind's Eye" and there were many practices devoted to the development and training of this organ. These training techniques involved the individual meditating with their eyes closed and focusing clearly on the Third, or minds, eye while adopting specific poses that were believed to help improve the "vibration" of the Third Eye, opening it with the aim of connecting with the same vibrations emanating from the universal energy field.

Images, Art and the Third Eye

Symbolism has been used throughout history to denote the Third Eye as a concept. In some representations the eye takes the form of exactly that, an eye placed in the center of the forehead. However, in many traditions a pine-cone has come to symbolize the Third Eye. This symbol can be found in many cultures, including that of Ancient Egypt. At first glance, with whichever eye you choose to use, this may seem an odd symbol and there is certainly something oddly coincidental about the choice of the pine-cone. The Pineal Gland, whether or not this was known to ancient cultures, is roughly the shape of a pine-cone (hence the name given to it by modern science. Whilst it's possible that in some cultures ancient pathologists or priests were aware of the shape of this gland it seems unlikely that all of the depictions are the result of dissections. Depictions of the Third Eye (or its equivalent) which illustrate it as a pine-cone can be found in cultures as diverse as Ancient Egypt, ancient Assyria, ancient Mexican cultures and the European Greek and Roman civilizations.

In all of these cultures the symbol appears to relate to both enlightenment and immortality. This latter seems to be a similar concept to that which Descartes later gave the Pineal Gland when describing it as the "seat of the soul". As a symbol, pine-cones are also interesting in that not only do the trees that bear them appear to be immortal, or evergreen, but also they are some of the most ancient surviving species of plant on the planet, predating flowering plants by many millennium.

The Links between the Pineal Gland and Third Eye

The Pineal Gland may also be referred to as the "pineal body" or the epiphysis cerebri. It is a simple, pea-sized structure but this small structure has some amazing qualities. The Pineal Gland produces several "chemicals" in the body and it is considered important by psychologists as these "natural happy drugs" can have a profound effect on both mood and on personality. Modern day theosophists, and those who study the esoteric, are also keen fans of the gland. For these groups it seems to provide a physical manifestation within the brain of the ancient concept of the Third Eye. For this group it is considered to be the most powerful source of energy and enlightenment that we possess and also responsible for psychic abilities of every kind. This group also argue that a closed Third Eye is responsible for negative emotions, including cynicism, anger, envy and lack of belief (in both the spiritual and the self). This argument has plenty of basis in fact, given that without a fully functioning Pineal Gland, the chemicals our bodies need to regulate mood, in a positive way, are absent.

The Third Eye is viewed as a gateway to developing and improving our psychic abilities and helps to improve the performance of our Sixth Chakra. Opening the Third Eye and bringing the Sixth Chakra to its fullest potential are often equated with the skills of the psychic and the clairvoyant. Active, and well developed, the Pineal Gland appears to promote both creativity, imagination and also to help to remember our dreams more clearly. It has also been linked to the ability to control our dreams (known as lucid dreaming) and to awake, or develop, precognition in many different forms. The Pineal Gland does, in fact, seem to become active during the night, particularly at the times when we normally dream. Usually, our dreams are at their most active between 01:00 am and 16:00 am and the Pineal Gland has been observed to become most active in average individuals at this time.

Science and Hallucinogenic Drugs

When it comes to natural “happy drugs” there's a lot of dispute about the role that the Pineal Gland plays. While it is well established that the gland is responsible for the production of melatonin, recent research suggests that it may well be secretly supplying a more hard-core drug to our system. The drug in question is “dimethyltryptamine”, and it appears that the Pineal Gland may be able to secrete this hallucinogenic naturally in the body. In recent years the drug has been found to be present in a wide range of both plant and animal species. Its natural production in humans is now established, but the purpose, the amounts and the "why" is as yet unclear.

Some researchers believe that the drug can (and does) flood the body during the process of birth and also that of death. Additionally there have been suggestions that this natural drug is present in the body during the 13th week of pregnancy, although clear evidence of this is yet to be fully established. If this latter fact is true, another strange coincidence with ancient teachings may be found in relation to the Pineal Gland – the 13th week of pregnancy is traditionally considered in Tibetan Buddhism to be the point at which the soul enters the physical body!

Scientifically, the Pineal Gland is, in fact, a real "Third" eye; the tissues from which it is formed are the same as those from which the retina is composed. As in animals which have a more clearly defined Third Eye the Pineal Gland remains sensitive to light in humans and although the mechanism of how this works is not fully understood, scientists have established that light levels have a direct impact on this small, deeply hidden gland!

The Faulty Third Eye Dilemma

We all have a Pineal Gland and the chances are that yours is working! Certainly it would be impossible to sleep at all (ever) if the Pineal Gland we possess was not functioning. Although some people suffer from insomnia from time to time, the condition is nearly always related to other health problems or results from issues not related to the Pineal Gland. In most individuals the Pineal Gland is fine! However, some people seem to possess psychic and clairvoyant qualities naturally, or have learned to "open" their Third Eye effectively. While everybody has a Pineal Gland, not everybody appears to have psychic abilities.

As mentioned earlier in this book, the Pineal Gland is one of those parts of the body that is sensitive to calcium deposits. This process, calcification, can happen in soft tissue in different parts of the body but is most commonly seen in arteries, heart valves and the Pineal Gland itself. The condition is caused by imbalances in vital vitamins (vitamin K2 deficiency and vitamin D overdose) and these imbalances can alter the way in which our body absorbs calcium (essential for bone development) and allow deposits to accumulate in the wrong areas.

Unfortunately modern lifestyles and our modern diet are not, despite what we may believe, what we were built for. Our bodies, including that small pea-sized gland, have evolved over tens of thousands of years and have not adapted for either the way in which we now live or the food that we commonly eat. This, in turn, means that both our lifestyle and diet can lead to poor nutrition and general health, and these factors greatly increase the risk of calcification. Although this calcification is actually a natural part of the aging process, calcification of the Pineal Gland seems to happen disproportionately early and is common by our teenage years, developing to a much greater extent by the time we are only in our forties. In some cases the gland simply begins to shrivel and wither away, retaining limited function in either its physical or psychic senses. This goes a long way towards explaining why so many people believe that they are not (or could not be) psychic in anyway. There is, however, some good news; opening your Third Eye and de-calcifying your Pineal Gland are perfectly possible! In the rest of this book we'll explore the best techniques to achieving exactly that!

Chapter 3: De-calcifying the Pineal Gland

The Pineal Gland is not, as we've seen, some esoteric, hard to define, otherworldly concept. It's real, it's pea-sized and it's located directly between the two sides of your brain. As part of our body it is directly affected by what we put into that body in the form of food, drink and chemicals of all kinds. As we saw earlier in the book the Pineal Gland is not protected by the "brain-blood-barrier" which inhibits harmful elements flowing directly to our brain. This is part of the reason why the gland is more susceptible to what we eat, drink and ingest than the rest of our brain. While our brain does need some very specific food types, to help it get the energy it needs to function, our Pineal Gland can be the most vulnerable part of the brain when it comes to the wrong kind of diet. In addition to diet there are some chemicals that we routinely ingest and these can be particularly harmful to our Pineal Gland. In this chapter we'll look at the practical steps you can take to de-calcify your Pineal Gland through your diet.

Fluoride and the Pineal Gland

Fluoride is present in our diets in surprisingly large amounts – it's naturally occurring and one of the important minerals we need. However, as with anything in life, it's possible to have too much of a good thing. Our modern diets are fluorinated to a startling extent; fluoride is added to our water, to toothpaste, to sodas, to processed foods and to canned foods. It's everywhere! Unfortunately, this overdose of fluoride means it makes its way to our Pineal Gland and it's one of the major causes of calcification in this part our body. The following steps should be taken to reduce your fluoride intake to a natural amount.

- Tap water is usually fluorinated and it's important to avoid this in order to de-calcify your Pineal Gland. Use a water filter or buy purified, distilled water.

- Toothpaste is the next big source of over-kill on the fluoride front. Increasingly, as we become more concerned about our health in general, it's far easier to buy low fluoride varieties – or better still those with no fluoride at all.

- Avoid red meat (occasional amounts are OK and should be part of your diet) and any and all processed foods that you can.

- Try to eat only organic fruit and vegetables. The non-organic variety contain a cocktail of drugs and chemicals, many of which are harmful to your health in general.

While some of these steps may be relatively easy, some may take some time to adopt and incorporate into your lifestyle. Persevere until you are, mostly, avoiding the most harmful of these. The benefits will begin to become apparent as your Pineal Gland opens and your Third Eye activates. However, while the psychic benefits are great, the real physical benefits that you'll reap in terms of better health and resistance to illness and infection are worth the effort on their own!

Supplements That Can Help

In addition to foods and products to avoid, there are several dietary supplements that will help to speed the process of de-calcifying your Pineal Gland. These are listed below.

- Iodine; supplements containing iodine help to reduce high levels of fluoride in the body. As a supplement this is great for your health, as it moderates the amount of fluoride in your system (we do need some). It can also help to ensure that your de-calcified Pineal Gland is not subject to further deposits.

- Tamarind; this food is good for your de-calcification as it helps, as with iodine supplements, to reduce fluoride levels in the body. However, it seems particularly to have an effect on the Pineal Gland, helping to block deposits of calcium.

- Cod Liver Oil; good for the body and, it seems, the mind. This product contains high levels of Omega 3, a natural fatty acid, which is important for keeping your joints supple and is also an essential "brain-food". This supplement will ensure a healthy body and a healthy brain, including your Pineal Gland.

- Bentonite Clay; this is a good detox supplement which removes chemicals and heavy metals from your system. As the Pineal Gland is more at risk from contamination by these than other parts of the brain it's a great supplement to consider.

- Ginseng; again this is a popular detox supplement and can be simply drunk in the form of tea. It helps to remove toxins from the body (benefiting the Pineal Gland) and it also is known to increase the function of the immune system, giving an all-round health boost.

- Melatonin; this is the hormone produced by the Pineal Gland itself and it can be severely affected by calcification. Low levels of melatonin can lead to chronic depression, fatigue and anxiety issues. Melatonin supplements will boost your mental state and help to encourage normal function in the Pineal Gland.

Traditional Techniques

In addition to these practical steps that will help you to decalcify your Pineal Gland, there are a number of alternative methods that you can use. These are based on traditional techniques used in a variety of traditions – some new, some old – to help re-activate or activate the Third Eye. These can be, possibly should be, used in conjunction with the steps above.

- Essential Oils; these can be used in your bath, on your pillow or during meditation (more on this later). Essential oils that have been traditionally associated with the Third Eye (Sixth Chakra) are; lavender, pine, frankincense and Davana oil.

- Turn off the Lights; the Pineal Gland is sensitive to light and darkness but the latter has been banished from our world almost completely by the widespread use of electric lighting! In fact, lights and screens of all kind mimic natural daylight, which effectively short-circuits our Pineal Gland. Learn to embrace the darkness in your life by turning off gadgets and any non-natural light source from time to time! Ideally, the last hour or so before bed should be natural light only. You can use candles or very low lighting (whichever is safest, most suitable and practical) but be sure to get away from the always-on approach on a daily basis.

- Linked to the above, is learning to allow your body to fall asleep and awaken naturally. This will help to re-adjust your natural body-clock which is regulated by the Pineal Gland. In addition to the above tip, practice waking up as it becomes light and allowing your body to gradually come round as it gets lighter.

- Chanting "Om" may sound an unlikely way in which to stimulate the Pineal Gland but modern science has discovered that the sound has a direct physical impact on the brain and the skull. It simply creates a real, physical vibration which, although the reasons are unclear as yet, helps to stimulate the Pineal Gland.

- Smart phones, or any wireless device emit electro-magnetic waves (EMF). These waves have been found to potentially cause damage to the Pineal Gland (and possibly other parts of the body and brain). Most of us cannot live without these devices today – but try to limit the time you spend with them.

- Crystal Healing; another ancient technique and one that has long held associations with the Chakras and re-balancing energy. In this case any crystal or precious stone colored purple is believed to help heal the Chakra and/or the Pineal Gland. These include purple sapphire, tourmaline and amethyst – though there are many others and choosing your favorite is no bad idea! We'll take a further more detailed look at crystal healing later in this book.

Chapter 4: Crystals and Meditation for the Third Eye

Crystal Healing is a whole subject in itself but in the context of this book we'll look at specific healing techniques which are recommended for opening the Third Eye and increasing your psychic abilities, along with your spiritual awareness. There are several books available on the subject of crystal healing in general and these may be useful tools to explore as you develop your abilities. For the time being, using the following techniques will help to open and heal your Third Eye.

Crystal Healing Basics

Different types of crystal vibrate with different frequencies of energy and these energies can also be found in each different Chakra. By using appropriate crystals you can help to strengthen this vibration and therefore activate your Third Eye. Stones that are suitable for the purpose include most gemstone (precious or semi-precious) that are colored purple. Several are mentioned in the previous chapter but Amethyst and Indigo are popular options and are widely available online or from New Age or spiritualist stores. The technique is simple; after cleansing and charging your crystal, you simply mentally focus on the crystal and "place" your intention within the stone and, when this is completed, place it in an appropriate location (or carry it with you). These basic steps are outlined below;

1. Cleansing your crystal; this should be done, ideally, in pure or distilled water with natural sea salt added to it. Leave the crystal submerged in the water overnight, for at least eight hours.

2. Charging your crystal; this is normally achieved by placing the crystal in direct sunlight for several hours. For the best effects place the crystal on a window which receives full sunlight (south facing) throughout the day. Although it's possible to leave the crystal for around five hours, the best results will be achieved by placing the crystal on the window as the sun rises and leaving it in place until sunset. Again, for the most powerful results, do this during summer, when the highest level of exposure to natural sunlight can be achieved.

3. Program your crystal; in a quiet place where you will not be disturbed, make yourself comfortable and lie back, flat on your back. Use a small pillow, if necessary, and then place the cleansed, charged crystal on your forehead, between, but a little above, your eyes.

Close your eyes and relax, focusing on your intention for the crystal. In this case, think about the purpose of the Third Eye. State the purpose you require of the crystal clearly; for example say “I wish to open my Third Eye”. Vary the statement as you see fit to include increasing your psychic abilities, your spiritual awareness or your clairvoyant skills. Be clear in your intention for the crystal and also keep the statement simple. Repeat the statement several times, keeping this up for a few minutes as a minimum is ideal and the longer the better!

4. Place your crystal appropriately; this is up to you, but many people will keep the crystal under their pillow, or close by in their bedroom. It's also common to carry the programmed crystal with you. This can be done in a pocket or a specially made bag. Neither method is preferable – choose which you feel comfortable with. Importantly, try to avoid crystals programmed for different purposes from touching each other, to avoid damaging the energy they emit.

Meditation and The Third Eye

Meditation is an ancient practice and forms an essential part of all major – and plenty of minor – spiritual practices. Prayer, reflexion and meditation can be found in as diverse a set of religions as it's possible to imagine. From Jain traditions (one of the oldest still practiced traditions in the world) to "younger" belief systems including Christianity and Islam. Wherever you look, meditation forms an aspect of both worship and spiritual discovery. It should be no surprise then, that it plays an important role in developing, opening and using your Third Eye! In this section we'll take a look at a simple meditation technique that will help you to develop your own Third Eye. For those that are unfamiliar with meditation techniques, we've structured the process in three steps, each building on the other and all working towards opening your Third Eye. Practice each section until you are proficient and then move on to add the next step.

Basic Meditation – Step 1 – Learning to Meditate

1. Create a quiet space to meditate, ensure you will not be disturbed by any intrusions, including excess noise and light. Wear comfortable clothing and ensure that the temperature in the room you are using is also comfortable, neither excessively warm nor cold.

2. Once you are settled comfortably (you can lie or sit, whichever is easier) begin breathing in a slow, deep and rhythmical way. To be sure that you are breathing in deeply enough, breathe through your stomach (pushing it out as you breathe in and contracting it as you breathe out). Count to four as you breathe in, hold your breath for two and count to four as you

breathe out. Breathe in through your nose and out through your mouth.

3. If you feel tension in any part of your body direct your breathing to that part; imagine the tension dispersing as you breathe out and feel each muscle relax. If you experience thoughts intruding on your meditation simply acknowledge them but don't dwell on them. Allow them to drift through your consciousness but don't stop to focus on any of them.

Basic Meditation - Step 2 - Locating the Third Eye

1. Once you have mastered basic meditation, described above, you can add the following stages to the process to begin to become aware of your Third Eye. Once you are in a meditative state begin to shift your focus from your breathing to your forehead; think of the feel of it, any wrinkles and the eye brows. Gradually focus on the point above the eyes and to the center of the forehead.

2. Now focus your breathing on this area; imagine energy being drawn into it as you breathe in and any negative energy being dispersed as you breathe out. Gradually you will feel a light tingling sensation in the area of the Third Eye, which indicates that it's awakening and that you have successfully located it.

Basic Meditation – Step 3 – Using a Mantra

1. Once you can regularly feel the presence of your Third Eye you can add a Mantra to your meditation. Specific mantras in the form of single sounds are associated with each of the Chakras; in this case the sound is "THOH". The word is pronounced as in "though" with the focus on the "th" sound. Tip: you can check online for audio clips of this Mantra to ensure you are pronouncing it correctly. Pronounce the word as you breathe out and try to extend it for as long as possible, take a pause, breathe in and then repeat as you breathe in. Repeat this for several minutes, or longer, and repeat the meditation every day for three to five days. You should begin to feel a clear tingling in the region of your Third Eye – and may initially experience this as a headache. This will pass and after a few days the sensation should feel pleasant and filled with energy.

2. After repeating the meditation with the Mantra until you can feel this sense of energy in the Third Eye, continue to meditate daily without using the Mantra. Simply breathe energy in to the Third Eye during meditations and expel any negative sensations. Gradually you will find that you experience very vivid dreams, flashes of prediction or psychic moments on

a regular basis, along with a deepened sense of intuition and a general rise in creative feelings or expression. At this point you can relax; you've successfully opened your Third Eye!

Chapter 5: Life With Three Eyes

Life with an open Third Eye is very different to life with just the "standard issue" two. In this final chapter we'll take a look at some of the changes – and the new experiences and sensations that you will begin to see appearing in your life.

An Eye in the Back of Your Head?

You may have heard the saying "they must have eyes in the back of their head" and when you have opened your Third Eye you may begin to see and experience the world in a whole new way. Intuitive abilities are often the first to develop as the complex relationship between our conscious and sub-conscious mind becomes more attuned. Our sub-conscious is the repository of all of our experience – many would argue both in this life and previous ones. When you have activated your Third Eye you have far greater access to this side of yourself and soon you'll see patterns in life, in events and in circumstances around and you'll be much quicker at seeing the most likely outcome of situations. Gradually this will build into truly "clairvoyant" abilities – the abilities to see so clearly that it seems – and may well be – that you can predict the future.

Meet The Ancestors

As your Third Eye heals and develops there is also a strong likelihood that your connection to, and ability to communicate with, the world of spirit will increase dramatically. We all have spirit guides and we are all influenced by the spirit world continuously. This normally manifests in most peoples' lives as simply being in the right place at the right time, or noticing some "uncanny" coincidences, which lead them to make a specific decision. With an active, healthy and fully functioning Third Eye, this communication will become more two-way and you may find that spirits will speak to you directly. This is often apparent at first, when you begin to sense close friends or family members who have passed away. In time, this sense will develop to include those who gather around other people, including complete strangers.

Strange Vibrations

Many people develop these in the early stages of decalcifying the Pineal Gland and opening their Third Eye. The most common sensations are a strong tingling in the area at the center of the forehead, where the Third Eye is traditionally depicted. For some this is a light, tickling sensation as if being brushed with a feather. For others, the feeling is of a constant, pressure or touch. In a minority of cases headaches or even migraines can occur. This is *rare* but does happen on occasion; headaches will pass in a few days, usually become less strong over that period. These sensations are widely documented and no cause for concern but simply a natural part of the process. The light tingling or touching sensation will usually pass after a few weeks – or at least become so familiar that it goes unnoticed. Some individuals find that during periods of insight, medium-ship or clairvoyance they notice or experience the sensation again. Many individuals with an active Third Eye take this to be an indication that there is a need to use the abilities (clairvoyance, medium-ship or spirit contact) as and when the sensation returns.

Living with the Dead

Death is not an end, simply a transition and a natural part of our spiritual journey. It's an inevitable part of opening your Third Eye that you will begin experience more contact with the world of spirit. In the early days after opening your Third Eye this contact will most often come in the form of dreams. Lost relatives or friends may appear in your dreams in a more vivid way than they have in the past. Conversations with them will seem more "real" in dreams and this is no coincidence! Listen carefully to what they say and be sure to consider any advice they give you. While spirits of all kinds have a more far-reaching view of our own world and lives, don't assume you must take all advice! Certainly the beings you find yourself in contact with are well informed but it's important to learn (or remember) to act using your own intellect and initiative and not come to rely on otherworldly advice.

Encountering spirits in dreams is common in the early stages of developing your Third Eye, but encountering them in the waking world is not uncommon and is increasingly likely as you develop your skills. Thanks to Hollywood, our impression of "ghosts" is largely negative and may leave you fearful for your safety. In reality, this impression is flawed; you're more likely to come to physical harm from a real person, in the real physical world, than you are from any spirit contacts you make. The physical realm is not the natural realm of spirit – it's yours! Remember this, and with this in mind, be aware that you can always ask unwanted, unwelcome or unhelpful spirits to leave. They have little choice but to do as you request and your intention is important here. Mean what you say and say what you mean when dealing with spirits of all kind. This works with people in our physical lives as well!

Heightened Sensitivity

This is an often overlooked issue for people dealing with their new skills. With an active, healthy Third Eye you will very quickly become more intuitive and extremely open to the emotions of the people around you. This can include complete strangers as you pass them on the street. Emotions are big things; they can be great and they can be terrible. Opening yourself up to them can leave you feeling drained and exhausted. You will certainly find that you'll be unwilling to spend time around those who emanate negative emotions and your sense of empathy will expand rapidly as you open your Third Eye. Empathy should not be confused with sympathy – you will feel what the person you are connecting with feels as if the feelings were your own.

As you take your first steps working with the Third Eye the best advice is to avoid those people or situations in which you are exposed to negative emotions. These will drain your energy and can leave you unable to work effectively with your Third Eye or enjoy the benefits of using it. However, as you become more experienced in life with three eyes, consider the benefits that your new "powers" can offer others. An important part of our spiritual growth is related to the way we interact with the world around us and, particularly, the way in which our actions to others are conducted. Using your "powers" or abilities to benefit only you will lead you to becoming small, narrow minded and selfish, which will ultimately destroy those powers! Learn to be strong and use your abilities of empathy to help, to heal and to benefit those around you. Importantly, remember to take time for yourself; walk in the woods and mountains alone, meditate, swim, and daydream. Whatever “re-charges” your batteries, ensure you make as much time for this as anything else; this will help to ensure that you have the reserves of strength to use your skills to their best effect.

Getting, or Staying, Physical

Many people have neglected their Third Eye for so long that opening it can be an astounding experience. It can become, almost, an obsession but remember that while it is massively important to your spiritual development you are not, as yet, pure spirit. We have real, urgent, physical needs in life; they're simple and include staying fit and healthy, eating well and socializing. All of these activities should be considered as cornerstones of your life. With an open Third Eye it is likely that you'll find that you are actually keen to eat and live healthily; go with that feeling! Learn to balance your physical, emotional and spiritual needs equally in life and make time for all three.

New Friends and Old

As your spiritual journey progresses you may find that some people in your life don't fit anymore. Don't be afraid of this – we all outgrow people from time to time. As your psychic and spiritual path progresses it's likely that you'll seek out new opportunities for learning and development and these will also bring new contacts into your life. Don't be afraid to let go of the past and explore the future in all areas of your life. This doesn't mean you should drop friends or associates lightly – you may have a deep bond with many of them and they may contribute to who you are in ways that you have yet to discover. However, if some contacts are lost as part of your journey learn to accept that this is part of the process.

Patience, Patience, Patience

Finally, be patient as you await the opening of your Third Eye. The steps and advice in this book will help to make the process real and viable but it can take more time for some than it can for others. For those already with a deeper spiritual awareness or natural clairvoyance the process can be rapid – days, weeks or a couple of months. For some, it can be lengthier, with progress and delays on the way. Remember to be patient and to persevere; you may need to make many changes in your life as your skills develop and some of these can take time and effort to achieve. The more times you try, the greater your chance of success and don't, whatever you do, be put off by occasional failures – pick yourself up and start again. You will get there!

Conclusion

Thank you again for reading this book!

I hope this book was able to help you to understand the facts and explode some myths behind the concept of the Third Eye and its relation to the Pineal Gland.

The next step is to try some of the steps suggested to de-calcify your Pineal Gland and begin the process of opening your own Third Eye. I hope the book will help with both and that you will soon begin to reap the full benefit of "life with three eyes"!

Finally, if you enjoyed this book, please take the time to share your thoughts and post a review on Amazon. It'd be greatly appreciated!

Thank you and good luck!

Preview of Chakras For Beginners

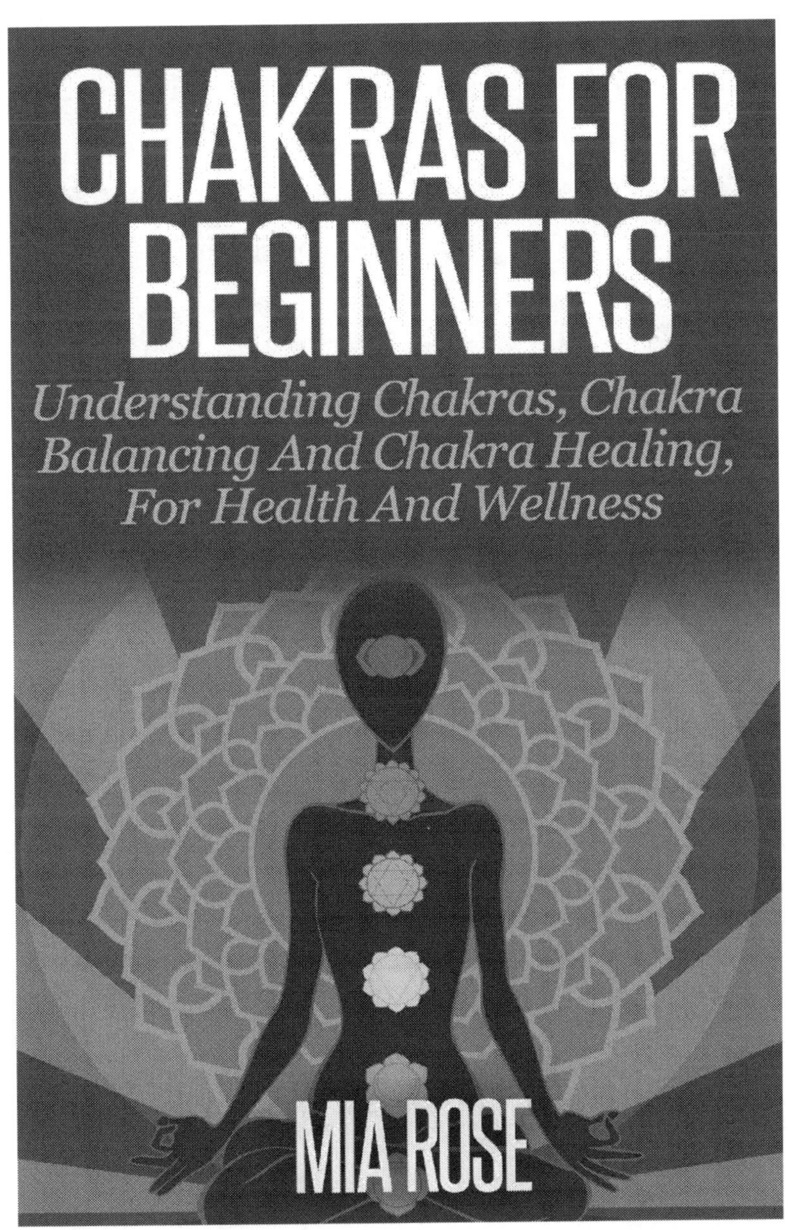

The ancient study of Chakras has made its way into the western world as of late. Frequently the first exposure can come through the study of yoga, meditation or Hindu practices.

The body and every living being is filled with a universal energy that connects and surrounds us. This energy can has been described as being made up of 7 layers (Auras) and the 7 chakras (energy points or knots in the body)

This book is designed to offer a practical, usable introduction to the Chakras, how they can affect our health and well-being and how to identify imbalances and address these.

The book is designed for those new to the concept but will also be useful for those with some experience of Chakra and energy healing. In the next chapter we take a more detailed look at what the Chakras are, and an overview of each one of the seven main Chakras. The remaining part of the book looks at each individual Chakra and how to examine the Chakra for imbalances. The final chapter provides a simple list-style section of tools that traditional (and modern) Chakra experts believe are useful in achieving balance within your Chakra energy system.

When our Chakras are in balance they allow energy to freely flow through our bodies and keep us revitalized, healthy and connected to the world around us. However, imbalances within the Chakra system can cause the energy to become blocked, leading to ill health both physical and emotional.

Here Is a Preview of What you'll Learn...

- History Of Chakras
- What Chakras Are
- In-depth Description Of Each Chakra
- Causes Of Chakra Imbalances
- Chakra Test
- How To Balance Each Chakra

Click here to check out the rest of Chakras for Beginners on Amazon.

Check Out My Other Books

Below you'll find some of my other popular books on Amazon and Kindle. Check them out by clicking on the images. Alternatively, you can visit my author page on Amazon here.

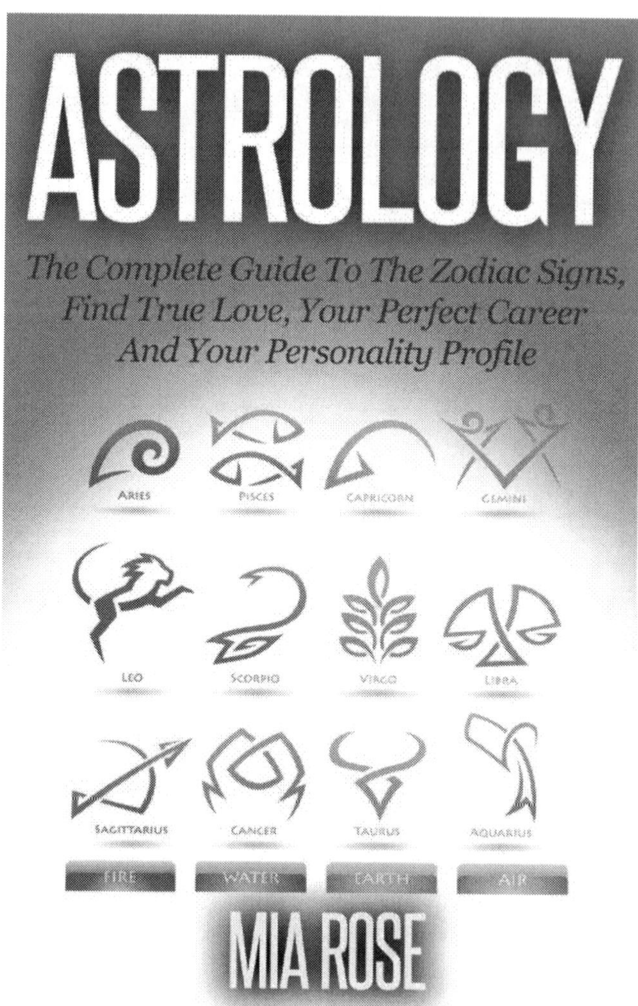

http://www.amazon.com/Astrology-Complete-Perfect-Personality-Horoscope-ebook/dp/B00N6HWV6K

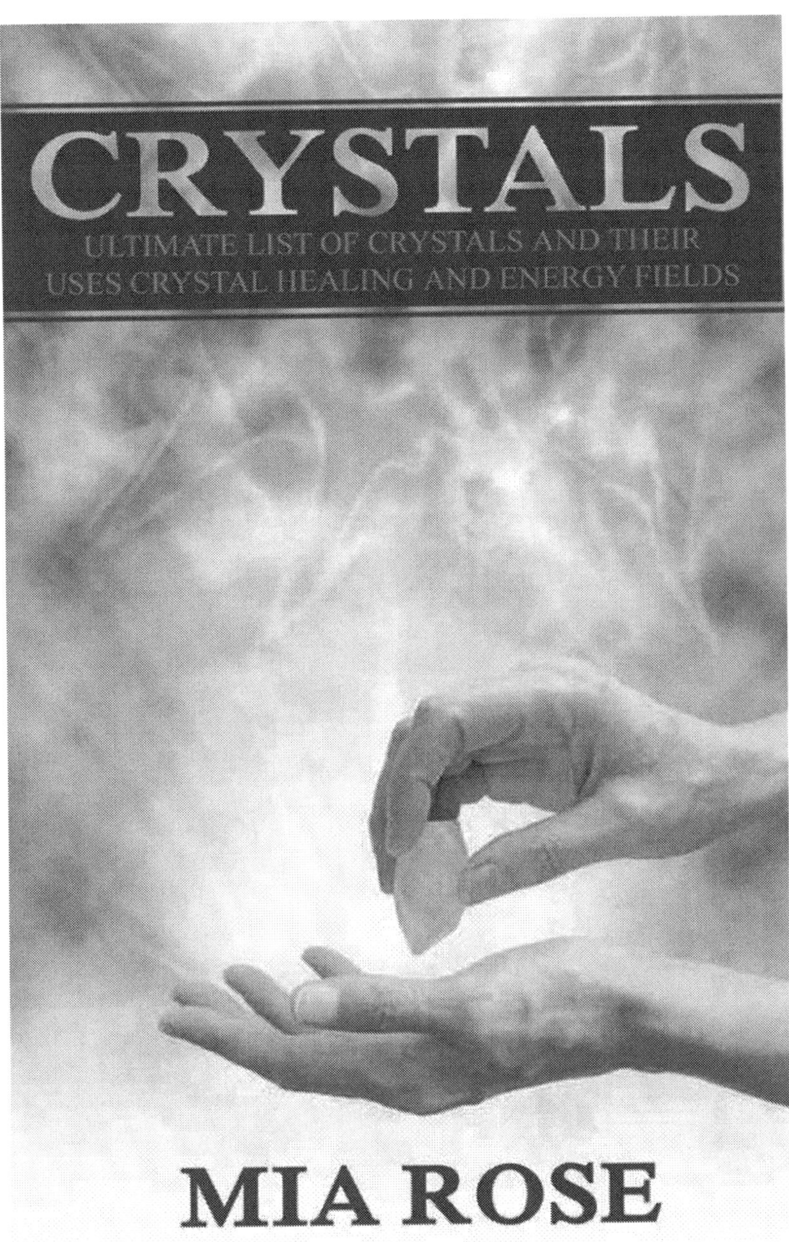

http://www.amazon.com/Crystals-Ultimate-Crystal-Healing-Spirituality-ebook/dp/B00SWMDP46

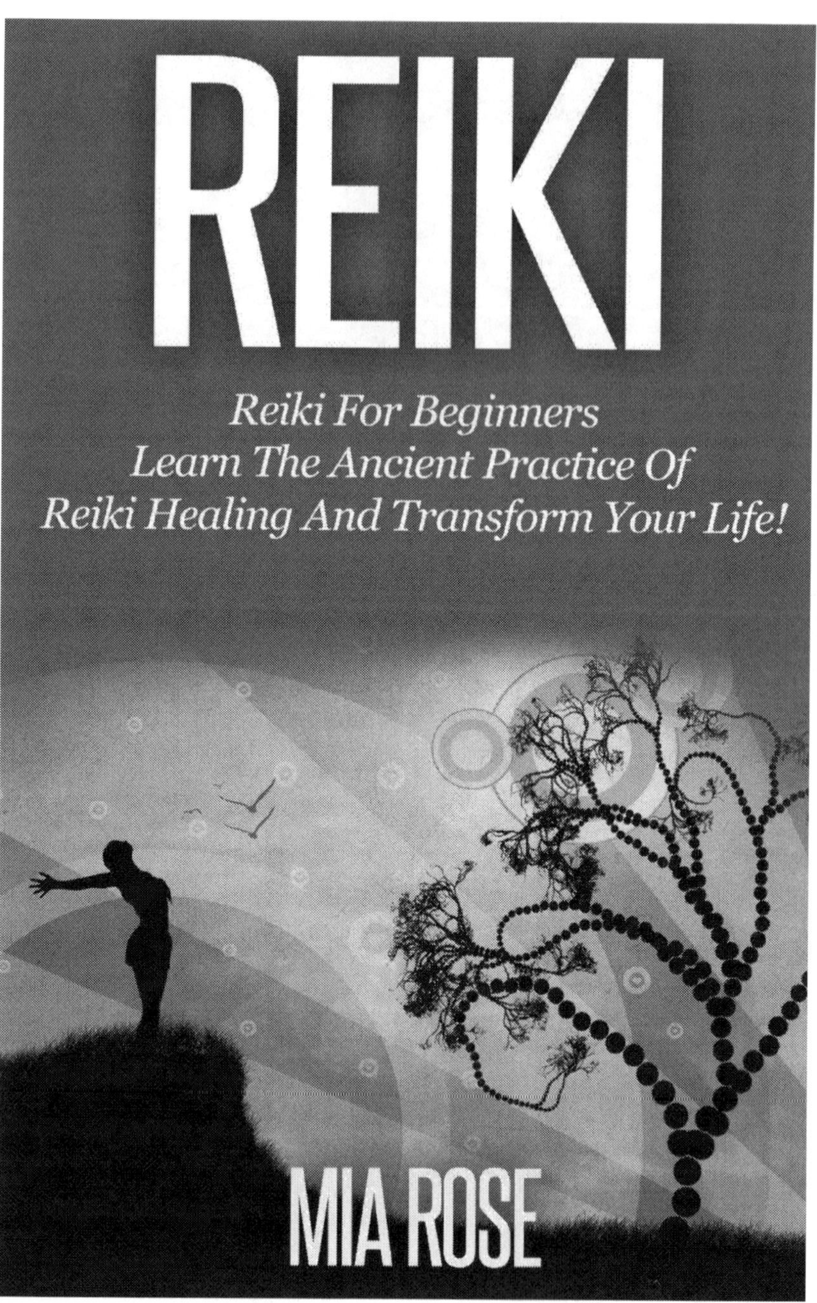

https://www.amazon.com/dp/1502391678

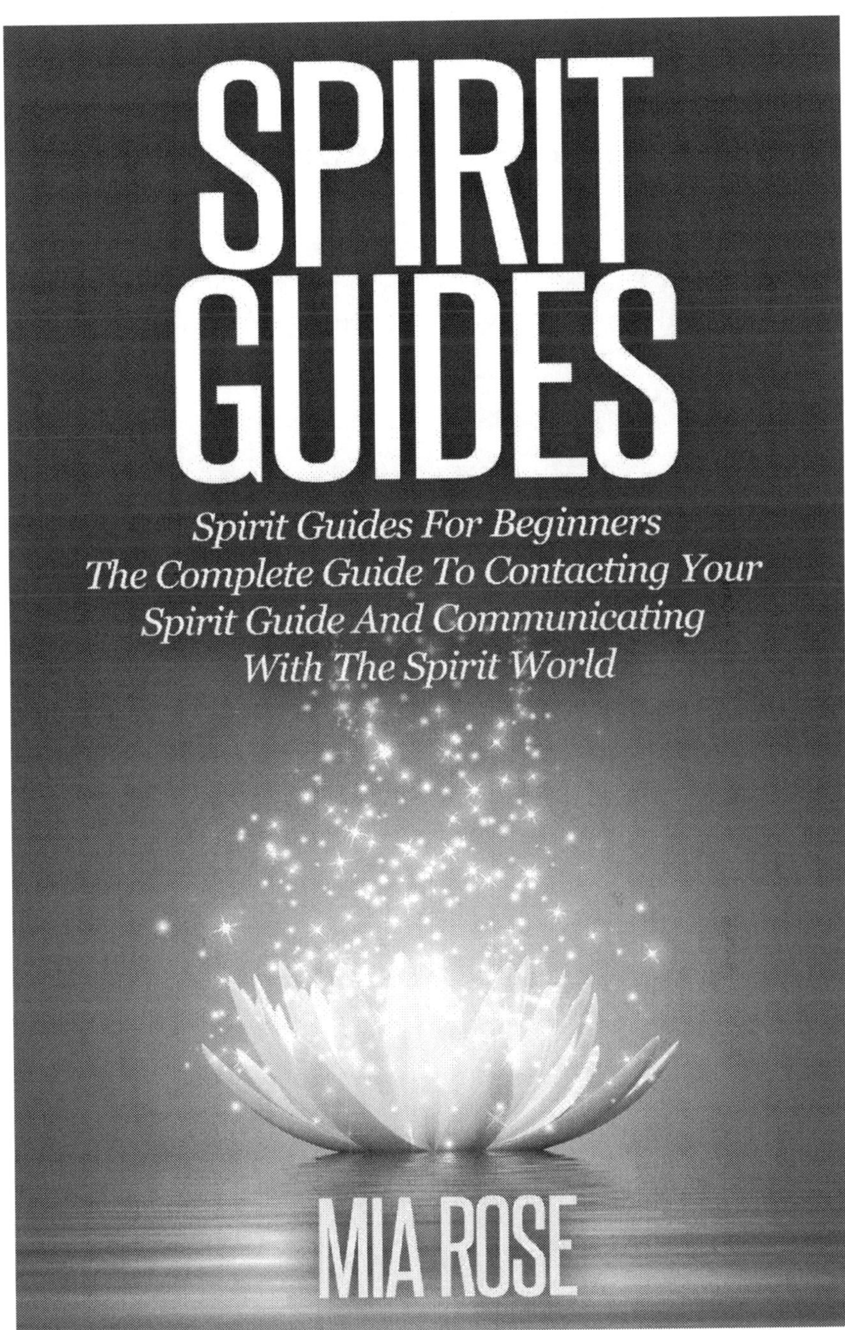

https://www.amazon.com/dp/1502502186

About the Author

I want to thank you for giving me the opportunity to spend some time with you!

For the last 10 years of my life I have studied, practiced and shared my love of spirituality and internal development. I kept diaries for years documenting the incredible changes that graced my life. This passion for writing has blossomed into a new chapter in my life where publishing books has become a full time career.

I feel extremely blessed and fortunate to have the opportunity to share my message with you! Each of my books are written to inspire others to explore the many aspects of their internal world. My goal is to touch the lives of others in a positive way and hopefully be the catalyst of positive change in this world :)

I am forever grateful for your support and I know you will get immense value through my books. I am really looking forward to serve you and give you great insight into my passions!

Your Friend

Mia Rose

Made in the USA
Middletown, DE
05 April 2024

52624931R10027